A SICK PREJUDICE

OVERCOMING OUR PRIMAL EMOTIONS AND
STEREOTYPES OF SOMEONE WITH A SERIOUS
ILLNESS

JOSEPH H. MCNOLTY

J.H.M.

JOSEPH H. MᶜNOLTY

Library of Congress-in-Publication Data

Edited by: Jennifer D. Munro

For more information about Joseph H. McNolty, visit: JosephMcNolty.com

For Ann

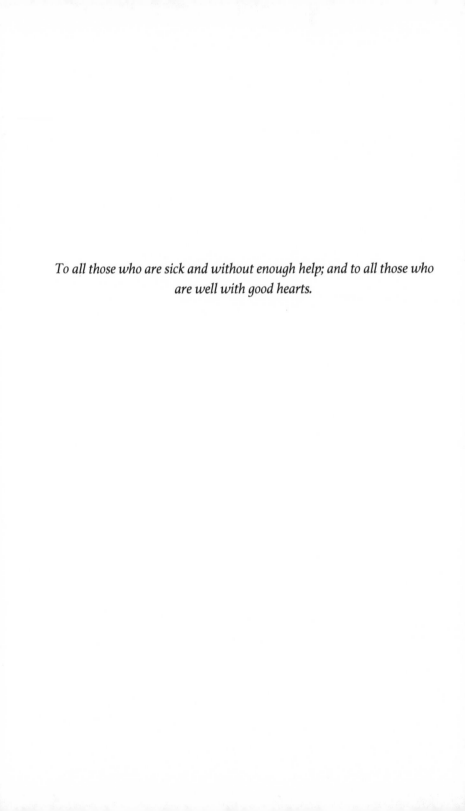

To all those who are sick and without enough help; and to all those who are well with good hearts.

CONTENTS

CHAPTER III. SICK PREJUDICE AVOIDANCE TACTICS THAT KEEP US FROM HELPING

CHAPTER IV. MANAGING A SICK PREJUDICE AND ENABLING A HEALING ENVIRONMENT

CHAPTER V. HELPING

CHAPTER VI. MOVING PAST OUR SICK PREJUDICE

PREFACE

What does "A Sick Prejudice" mean?

A sick prejudice means there are prejudgments made of people who have chronic, life-threatening illnesses. It means people have attitudes and assumptions already in mind when they go visit a sick friend or loved one. They don't view them or their illness as a unique circumstance. They see them through eyes that have been tainted by innate emotions, TV medical dramas, other sick people they've known, and how their families acted toward ill people. The book delves into how susceptible we are to feelings of a sick prejudice so we can understand and overcome them.

The biggest issue with an illness, as we learn, can be how people respond to it rather than the illness itself. For those of us who haven't had a serious illness, it's almost impossible to understand the changes it can have on the people around us, let alone ourselves. From one day to the next, a seriously ill person becomes a member of those who have some defect or disease. Just the word "disease" invokes feelings of fear and repulsion. All of a sudden, they're being treated like they *are* the disease.

Further, it's by their friends and loved ones during a time when the sick person is the most vulnerable. Worse yet, the sick one will likely have the same prejudices about sick people as everyone else and accept their bleak new role without question.

Why haven't we heard of "a sick prejudice" before?

A sick prejudice is mostly an invisible type of prejudice. People don't talk about it much; they don't talk about the stereotypes, biases, and assumptions we have about the chronically ill of our world. There isn't much in the news about how we interact with those having diseases and life-threatening illnesses. There are very few organizations representing and arguing on behalf of the seriously ill, unlike some other prejudices. Illness crosses all groups of people regardless of age, race, gender, ethnicity, religion, or political orientation, which makes the subject difficult to identify with. Lastly, it can seem self-betraying to talk of our true concerns and fears of sick people.

How is "a sick prejudice" like other prejudices?

A sick prejudice is like other prejudices in that conclusions are drawn about a person because they are in some particular group, such as a certain race, ethnicity or gender. A sick prejudice does an injustice to people who are seriously ill, just as racial prejudice does an injustice to people of color. A sick prejudice, however, doesn't have the animosity that racial prejudice can have. It's more about fear or apprehension, rather than dominance or hostility. A sick prejudice certainly has it's a harmful side though - it can make people sicker.

This book talks about how both a sick prejudice and racial prejudice likely began at the dawn of humanity, and are in some ways primitive, natural responses. In our modern world though, they are both useless and destructive. Of course, racial prejudices went on to become a great detriment in our society, causing years of oppression and miserable wars while sick prejudices, even at extremes, don't result in wars and violence, but rather the quiet abandonment of millions.

How large of a problem is "a sick prejudice"?

A sick prejudice appears to be a very large social and world problem. How large? We have a rough idea by using data from The Centers for Disease Control and Prevention. In 2012, they stated: "Approximately half of U.S. adults have at least one of the ten chronic conditions examined. Furthermore, one in four adults have multiple chronic conditions."[1] That's 64 million people in 2016 who had at least two chronic conditions (adjusting for the population increase from 2012). Using the same rough calculation, 1.4 billion people in the world would have had multiple chronic conditions. Nearly a billion and a half people rank up there with the largest ethnicities, races, and world religions. A sick prejudice deserves the same attention, concern, and level of action that we give other prejudices.

We can trust that most people with serious chronic conditions would benefit from some level of assistance, whether it's a few hours a week or much more. This book asserts that most chronically sick individuals will encounter people with deep, preconceived and pessimistic assumptions about their illness. This means that most sick people are spending life affected, to some degree, by a sick prejudice. These people are not getting the everyday maintenance and emotional support needed to live fully. What may be more concerning is that most of us will likely have some serious health problem in our lives and one day come face-to-face with: "*a sick prejudice.*"

What aspects of "A Sick Prejudice" is this book about?

The focus of this book is to simply enable people like you and me to feel better about helping a sick person. It doesn't try to solve the lofty problems of a sick prejudice in the world, but rather how we can get fulfillment from seeing a sick loved one on a regular basis. It's about how important our attitudes and expectations can be to their healing. Our first step is to think of someone we know who is sick, read the book, and enjoy helping them. If we're able to help and feel good about our assistance, a lot of the problem is solved.

INTRODUCTION

(It All Starts Here)

Someone close to you is suddenly sick, really sick, like with cancer, a heart condition, the aftermath of a stroke, multiple sclerosis, AIDS, or some other chronic illness. Of course, you're worried about them. More than that, you may at times be having feelings of anxiousness, despair, and disbelief. You're shaken up and having some trouble concentrating at work. This is how I felt when my wife was diagnosed with cancer, and how I continued to feel periodically over the almost twelve years that followed until she passed away. During that time and over the past five years with my own multiple myeloma blood cancer, I started to see how people behaved and responded to illness. I realized that I also had ways of thinking about seriously ill people that I hadn't been aware of. Those thoughts were determining how I felt and what I did or didn't do in the defining times of an illness.

Then, it struck me: "Oh my god, there's some kind of prejudice about sickness in us—A Sick Prejudice." I experienced a great deal during those fifteen years and began to understand and research the deep emotional patterns, assumptions, and biases people have around a serious illness. Through greater understanding and personal growth, I became more compassionate and released my expectations of other people. *When we can find our way past a sick prejudice, we give our sick loved one the chance to be someone unique and a better opportunity to heal. In the process, we give ourselves vital and enriching experiences, too.*

DEFINING A SICK PREJUDICE AND
GLIMPSING ITS REPERCUSSIONS

At first, our concern and alarm urges us to do something to help the sick one right away. Then, it often happens. We unwittingly develop what I call a "Sick Prejudice": when our assumptions, sickness stereotypes, and fears about serious illness create negative distortions about the sick person. These distortions can cause us to reduce the help we give or keep us from helping at all. Our strong, primeval fears of death and illness can make us want to avoid our sick friend or loved one. Fuel these fears with a mishmash of distressing memories of a dying relative, responses learned from our parents in childhood, hundreds of TV medical dramas we've seen, and pessimistic survival statistics we've heard about and we're emotionally charged up for the worst.

Very little of what we see is just this unique person today. We can overreact to a sickness situation as though everything is a life or death matter. It all combines to give us unnecessary confusion, distress, and conflict when we think about helping someone sick. These prejudices aren't malicious, like racial prejudice, but they are at least as undeserved and damaging. They're also quite natural and to be expected, as we'll see. That, however, doesn't make them any less hurtful for those who are sick or less destructive for our society.

Perhaps you don't know someone with a serious illness now, but it's very likely that a friend, parent, spouse, or relative will get sick at some point and you will have the opportunity to help. In 2012, the Centers for Disease Control and Prevention stated, "Approximately half (117 million) of U.S. adults have at least one of the ten chronic conditions examined. Furthermore, one in four adults have multiple chronic conditions."[1] That means that you can easily become one of the 21% of U.S. adults who helped another adult in the last year, according to a 2009 study from National Alliance for Caregiving and AARP.[2]

I certainly never expected to have a serious, chronic illness become a part of my life. Then came that morning on a camping trip, when my wife woke up and couldn't swallow, keep her eyes open, or breathe well from the myestinia gravis. We were thrust into the medical world and a new life for the next twelve years. Along the way, I realized my own sick prejudices and to see it in others time and time again. It's different for each person who experiences it, *but it still all boils down to an emotionally distorted, exaggerated, and despairing outlook on illness for many potential helpers.* For many, it blocks their ability to freely help. For me, it blocked my ability fully to enjoy the remaining time I had with my wife by making the experience worrisome and stressful.

How we handle our helping role can impact the patient's survival rates and quality of life. Research from Johns Hopkins Center found that the support of family or friends has been shown to lessen the chance that one will become sick or die from heart disease. Other research conducted at Brigham Young University and the University of North Carolina showed that people who did not have strong social support were 50% more likely to die from illness than those who had such support.[3]

Even when we do dive in to help, the stereotypes and exaggerated feelings of a sick prejudice can keep us from having a rewarding and satisfying experience supporting our friend or family member. They are an undermining, corrosive influence on an illness situation. In the weeks and months that follow hearing about the illness, our sick prejudice can cause us to become cautious, dispassionate, and negative in our approach to the sick one. We start to feel an exaggerated sense of burden by them and the help they need.

It's as though the illness becomes an invisible, emotional sunburn for us. Like cringing when we're patted on a sunburned shoulder, we pull away from things we wouldn't have noticed or might have even enjoyed with the person before. We notice their faults and are more sensitive to how they talk to us. For example, we might think, "Gosh, they're complaining about everything." Before the illness, complaining might have been mutual and part of a lively, fun banter. Now, the playful nature and banter are lost. In their place are dread, fear, and sadness. We become more conscious of the "favors" we're doing for them, and may start thinking, "Are they taking for granted that I'm going to help? Is this going to be an everyday thing?" Making matters worse, it can seem "socially undesirable" or insensitive to talk about our deep feelings around illness.

Our sick prejudice fears and avoidance tactics may surface in a variety of thoughts and excuses:

1. "So and so had a horrible illness like this and then died. It was awful." (Assuming past experiences will be true now)

2. "I read they only have a 20% chance of beating this. It's so sad." (Assuming statistics are true)

3. "I'd like to help some, but if I start, will I get asked to do more than I want?" (Fear of losing control)

4. "Oh, god, what if they ask for money?" (Fear of burden)

5. "Now that I think about it, I don't even have a very close relationship with them." (Cutting emotional cords)

6. "They probably brought this on themselves by always..." (Basing help on perceptions of cause)

7. "They must have someone else who can help, someone not as busy as I am." (Getting Out/Bargaining)

8. "I don't want to bother them. I'll just let them know to ask if they ever need anything." (Avoidance)

In the later stages of a sick prejudice, our outlook can become unhappy and burdened, until we feel drained and start looking for ways to distract ourselves and forget about the situation. Ironically, our heightened concern and worry can become an obstacle to our continued friendship and love with someone who is very dear to us. Our stereotypes, assumptions, and primitive fears can shift our focus from how we used to see them to how we see them now that they have a chronic illness.

Symptoms of a sick prejudice can also cause responses of overconcern, desperation, and heightened busyness in the illness situation for those who already have empathetic, giving-type personalities. I am naturally empathetic. My assumptions, sickness stereotypes, and heavy online research about my wife's illness made for some miserable evenings around the house. Few or none of the outcomes that I tormented myself about ever happened. Fortunately, she remained lighthearted through most of her treatment, and I learned an old lesson: "It's not what happens, but how one thinks about what happens that matters" (Epictetus 55–135 AD).[4]

When my wife was first diagnosed with cancer in mid-2002 with thymoma cancer and myestinia gravis, I didn't realize then that I started seeing her through a mishmash of cancer stories, hospital shows, past sick relatives, cancer statistics, and primordial emotions about sickness. I was overcome at times with fear and dread, yet nothing other than a diagnosis had happened yet. My fear translated into worst-case scenarios that ranged from her dying soon, our health insurance not paying, to the loss of my career. *(The allure of what can go wrong can be immensely seductive.)*

Through my wife's cancer and then my own, I saw that anyone can "click" into sick-prejudice mode at any time, including family and myself. I eventually realized that the feelings and responses we have to illness are natural. That we're not selfish, uncaring, or cold, but rather responding in predetermined ways that unfortunately no longer serve us. Even though natural, the effects of a sick prejudice can be both harsh and unnecessary. Those effects sit squarely in the way of meeting two crucial objectives in a sickness situation:

1. to better enable the recovery of the sick one through our involvement as helpers, and

2. to make our helping experience fulfilling and sustainable for us.

When either of these objectives are not met, our sick friend or loved one may get sicker, and we lose meaningful life opportunities as potential helpers.

Isn't it hardest when it's our child, spouse, parent, or sibling who is sick? *The greater our love, the more heightened our ancient emotions can be, and the more unbearable it is to imagine them suffering and wasting away. Ironically, we may pull away from those we love most in their time of greatest need.* More unfortunate is that the unique way our loved one goes through a sickness will likely be nothing like our imaginings and nightmarish scenarios. We then can miss the opportunity to help them and feel good about ourselves, for reasons that aren't even true!

CHAPTER I. EXPLAINING WHY WE HAVE A SICK PREJUDICE

PART A. EVOLUTIONARY CAUSES OF A SICK PREJUDICE (AND SIMILARITIES OF A SICK PREJUDICE TO RACIAL PREJUDICE)

We have primitive emotions and impulses triggered by sickness that hover below our conscious, logical, thinking minds. The emotions can be stimulated directly from biological responses and specialized neural mechanisms in our body.[5] *That makes the idea of a serious illness in someone close to us not just a thought in our mind, but something we feel in our bodies.* These biological mechanisms can cause us to respond like a reflex, without even thinking. Controlling these reflexive feelings and impulses was extremely difficult for me. I'd seamlessly slip into an anxious, troubled state at the thought of a change in my wife's condition or one of her test results.

Based on the book *Evolution of Sickness and Healing*, by Horacio Fábrega, Jr., MD,[6] major sicknesses, diseases, or injuries are different from other kinds of stressors and problems in our lives because we have strong, primitive emotions about sickness and the pain that often accompanies it. The book exhaustively researches and extrapolates how evolution has formed innate human responses and behaviors around sickness and healing. The writing of *A Sick Prejudice* takes findings from Dr. Fábrega's work and further suggests that our subliminal interpretation of these primitive emotions can, in part, determine how we react to someone with a serious illness and whether we choose to help.

Our emotions around sickness are complex and can seem to contradict one another. Often, we feel compassion, caring, and a desire to help someone with a serious illness. In other cases, we feel a sense of dread, urgency and apprehension (Fábrega). We may evolve during our lives from more fear-based to more caring-based reactions, or vice versa. Different people may experience these dynamics in different ways.

The large part of the sick prejudice problem appears to arise when we interpret our strong biological and neurological responses to sickness and pain (Fabrega, 86–87) in fear and dread-filled ways, rather than in compassionate and empathetic ways. Our emotional experience is that something bad is happening and we may be in danger somehow. Negative feelings like these can cause us to withdraw from the emotionally charged situations of a serious illness. The important point is that it's evident that fear and avoidance-based reactions to seriously ill people do exist. These responses have detrimental consequences for the sick and debilitated, those around them, and society as a whole.

The chain reaction from primitive emotions to avoidance of an illness situation is the first part of a sick prejudice. We are prejudiced in that our reaction to our sick friend or loved one can be based on feelings and assumptions that have little or nothing to do with them individually, and we may take actions on those feelings, which make it harder for the sick one to recover or heal.

1. Our Deep Past

We are behaving in some ways based on emotional responses prompted from a drastically different time than today and projecting our expectations onto our ill friend or family member. Let's look more closely at why these primordial emotions are so deeply ingrained. Our adaptations and responses to sickness were "forged" throughout the often harsh and migratory conditions of the Pleistocene Epoch (2.6 million to 11,700 years ago) (Fábrega, 212–213).

Our human ancestors lived in conditions that at times were harsh, agonizing, and filled with frequent pain and suffering (Fábrega, 50). A serious infection or injury was often a death sentence (Fábrega, 50) that stimulated worry, fear, and strong emotions (Fábrega, 75). "The social and emotional atmosphere of healing for serious/protracted sickness was shrouded in ambiguity, concern, and potential danger...." There were "...crisis, life/death, and menacing implications of sickness and healing" (Fábrega, 107). Not surprisingly then, sickness was probably very disruptive within our small family-level groups (Fábrega, 80–89). How these emotions get translated into behavior is thought to have been complex, ranging from empathy and caring, to being ignored and abandonment (Fábrega).

As hunter/gatherers, we collected what we needed and at times struggled to find enough food for survival. Imagine when someone in a group got seriously sick or injured. It could've resulted in agonizing decisions (Fábrega, 90), such as whether to feed the sick person when there might be too little food already and now possibly fewer providers (Fábrega, 92). The group could feed the sick one out of attachment and sorrow, only to have them die anyway, reducing the group's strength in the process. Caring for the sick member could jeopardize the rest of the group in lean times and cold winters. (Do people today unnecessarily start emotionally disconnecting from a person?)

Our great ancestors were often on foraging expeditions, traveling in open country looking for food (Fábrega). If someone got very sick or injured, it could have been burdensome to carry them. They could already be half starved and now be unable to keep up with the animal herds they relied on, or get to the food sources they traveled to. *Imagine the emotional distress of having to leave a sick loved one behind in the middle of unfamiliar land with predators lurking, or possibly killing them so they didn't suffer* (Fábrega, 51)! Our survival at times would have depended on being dispassionate and breaking ourselves from attachment when someone got seriously ill or disabled. At some point, we would have had to decide whether the disabled one was too old, injured, or sick to be worth it. (Do people today needlessly judge the worth and usefulness of those with chronic illnesses (Fábrega, 84)?)

It's likely that these very early Homo sapiens held superstitions that illness was caused by evil spirits invading the sick one, by the gods being angry, or by the evil intentions of hostile neighboring groups (Fábrega). In addition, there was likely confusion around what was contagious both physically and spiritually, further scaring the others and isolating the sick one. There might have been stories passed down for generations about groups being decimated by something contagious. (Do people today still have superstitions or "illness phobias" to varying degrees when around an ill person?)

We would have experienced births, ate, slept, and died only a few feet apart in the close quarters of the family-level groups we lived in during this Pleistocene period. The physical bonding and emotional attachment from this intimate living would have magnified all the sounds of pain and sights of suffering of anyone sick or injured (Fábrega, 80–83).

This long evolutionary exposure to the deeply emotional and impactful consequences of sickness and disability by our human ancestors left lasting psychological and biological imprints in us (Fábrega, 214–216). Undoubtedly, our emotions have continued to evolve, but for roughly 99% of our evolution from Hominin to Human (i.e., Pleistocene Epoch 2.6 million to 11,700 years ago), serious sickness likely evoked fear and hardship.[7] This was when our basic human emotions and responses were embedded in our brains and bodies.

Even in more recent history, such as the Middle Ages, sickness had potentially devastating consequences to a family's livelihood and emotional stability. It would have been accompanied by confusion, distress, and tormented decisions of what to do amid false remedies and speculation. Black Death killed half of England's population by 1350.[8] Superstitions were rampant, ranging from sickness caused by sins to diagnoses based on astrology and planetary positions. The stories of measles, typhus, leprosy, small pox, dysentery, tuberculosis, and others likely contributed ample terror to the meaning of sickness. The dire specter of illness and disease has tormented humanity throughout its existence.

We've seen astounding advancements in healthcare in just the last 100 years, and geometrically in the last 50 years. The incredible advancements in medicine, surgery, and healing, coupled with the dramatic rise in our standard of living has fundamentally changed what major illness means. *Progress has been too fast and recent for our attitudes and emotions to have caught up. We're left clinging to the menacing fossils of what illness once meant.*

2. Similarities of Sick Prejudice to Racial Prejudice

In some ways, our learned evolutionary responses to sickness are a similar condition to those of racial prejudice. A 2005 Science-Daily article states, "Contrary to what most people believe, the tendency to be prejudiced is a form of common sense, hard-wired into the human brain through evolution as an adaptive response to protect our prehistoric ancestors from danger...because human survival was based on group living, 'outsiders' were viewed as— and often were—very real threats."[9]

Even with our conscious awareness of racism and best attempts at overcoming it, our "Implicit Biases"[10] sometimes cause us to respond in prejudiced ways. Implicit biases regarding race, gender, disability, body type, and others have been found in most of us. In an FAQ called "Helping Courts Address Implicit Bias," the National Center for State Courts (2012) defined implicit biases this way: "Unlike explicit bias (which reflects the attitudes or beliefs that one endorses at a conscious level), implicit bias is the bias in judgment and/or behavior that results from subtle cognitive processes (e.g., implicit attitudes and implicit stereo-types) that often operate at a level below conscious awareness and without intentional control."[11]

These innate racial tendencies have become a great detriment to our society causing thousands of years of oppression and wars. Likewise, our responses and emotions around sickness had very real causes for developing and are arguably more deeply entrenched in our minds than racial and other prejudices, due to the physical pain aspects of sickness. Our sick prejudices, though, are harder to see, because there isn't much in the news about the feelings and triggers around illness, unlike racial and gender prejudice. Also, life-threatening sicknesses cross all demographic groups (e.g., age, ethnicity, income, gender). *Even at extremes, sick prejudices don't result in wars and violence, but rather the quiet abandonment of millions.*

3. Summing Up: Sick-Prejudice Feelings are Natural but No Longer Relevant

We can see why news of a serious illness would trigger ancient, exaggerated feelings of concern and urgency.[12] *At a fundamental level, we may feel that something bad can happen to us if we get involved in a situation involving illness.* There can even be natural feelings of repulsion to sick people, to being in their homes, and going to hospitals. We can see now that our seemingly insensitive feelings of self-preservation, to pull back from a sickness situation at times, are perfectly natural.

A large part of a sick prejudice is about the distortions and ancient assumptions we have about someone with a life-threatening sickness, and NOT about us being inherently uncaring. We should expect to feel the symptoms of a sick prejudice and not try to deny the emotions and thoughts we have. While it's natural and understandable that most of us carry some form of a sick prejudice, it still causes unnecessary suffering for the sick and loss of meaning and growth for those around them.

It should be encouraging to know that we have innate drives and emotions to feel empathy, provide care, and make allowances in our daily lives for the sick. A hallmark of humanity is the medical structure we've created for healing and treating the sick. Medicines, hospitals, and physicians are an everyday part of life. The science we have developed in imaging technologies, pathology, cardiology, hematology, anatomy, and hundreds more testifies to the intentions we have to heal the sick. When it comes to our own involvement, however, our intentions can become conflicted with our "sick prejudices (Please see Figure 1)."

Figure 1
CONTINUUM OF REACTIONS TO A SERIOUSLY ILL PERSON
AND SICKNESS SITUATION

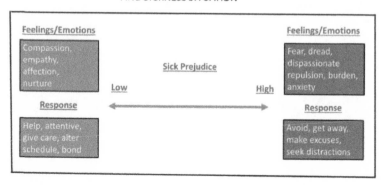

Most of us will encounter some serious illness in our lives, and for us to be responding from ancient internal programming is a drain on the well-being and prosperity of us all. *It keeps us from enjoying the fulfillment of being of service; it breaks the need-help-need cycle that we ultimately all flow through during our lives; it increases suffering, and it can shift burdens to social welfare systems that are economically less efficient and much colder in their delivery than we can be.*

PART B. RELIANCE ON PERSONAL EXPERIENCE CONTRIBUTES TO A SICK PREJUDICE

Our innate programming, anxiety, sense of dread, and implicit biases were probably reinforced as children when our parents fearfully reacted to news of major illnesses. Here's an especially appropriate quote: "Conversely, other types of developmental experiences may culminate in a tendency to minimize or withdraw from the effects of disease and injury in others. These are individuals who shun, avoid, or are repelled by disease and injury in others, which leads them away from a healing role"[13]

I vaguely remember it happening this way for me: My mother was on the phone with a newly diagnosed sick friend and exclaimed, "Oh, my God! That's terrible. I'm so sorry." Her voice filled the house with feelings of catastrophe and deep remorse. Later, when she talked in muffled tones with my father, I could see their lips tighten, eyes intensify, and voices become deadly serious. Like most children, I would have latched on to this scene with my perceptive young mind. Early childhood experiences like these could activate the underlying primitive impulses that we all have, predisposing us to react similarly when we hear about illnesses later in life.[14] I probably played out the role of my mother in very similar ways when I first got news of my wife's cancer diagnosis.

We rely on our own limited personal experience and general information about illness when someone close to us comes down with a chronic illness. We naturally reflect on any experiences we've had, stories we've heard, and TV shows we've seen. We assume the current situation could be like those and look for similarities that validate what we expect. Again, we project our expectations onto this situation. It's natural to look back on our experiences, but that doesn't mean they are accurate.

In my wife's case, I didn't fully recognize that the doctors, medicines, support systems, and type of cancer were all completely different than when my mother had breast cancer in the 1960s and later lymphoma in the 1980s. The closeness of a cancer experience with my mother's experience overwhelmed my judgment, as family illnesses often do. Nor did I appreciate that my wife and mother were two totally different people. The chemo my mother had for lymphoma made her very sick for eight months in classic chemo style for that time. My wife's chemo and radiation were dramatically better. Before I realized this, I brought lots of unnecessary stress onto myself and the situation from bringing the past into the present.

We've been taught that serious illness in the family is supposed to be emotionally trying and deeply worrisome. I learned that role well. The information I had was that serious illness takes a great toll on those around it. When my wife first became sick, I was overwhelmed with thoughts of, "How will I cope with this along with all of my other responsibilities?" My wife did need chemo, then open chest surgery to remove tumors, and finally radiation to remove any tidbits of cancer that remained. That was a touch-and-go process: lots of concern and sleeplessness for me about that, too. This was the most difficult time of my life, and even as a slender man, I lost about fifteen pounds in six weeks. She recovered nicely. All the worry and crafting of future scenarios on my part were unneeded and exhausting. To my relief, I found that all the problems broke down into logistics to be done one at a time. There simply wasn't the upheaval I expected. As Søren Kierkegaard is generally credited with saying, "The most painful state of being is remembering the future, particularly the one you'll never have."[15]

Time and again through my wife's twelve-year illness, I would slip into my ancient fears and projections of my mother with cancer only to have them proven wrong nearly every time. I didn't realize I was thinking about the past so I couldn't question the resulting feelings. The chores got done, meals got cooked, kids did their homework, I went to work, and I still did most of the things I had done before she got sick.

With such results, one would rationally start expecting positive outcomes, but the emotional weightiness of my past illness experiences kept my sick prejudices circling back. The result was incredibly stressful and worrisome times that were unnecessary and unhealthy for everyone.

When my time came, I was still suffering from a sick prejudice. I of course thought most about the cases that were closest to me—my wife and mother. Intellectually, I knew from my wife's illness not to make assumptions and to stay positive. I also knew things were different thirty years ago with my mother. Still, I thought, "They had cancer, I have cancer, and look what happened to them."

My case was to be entirely different. I had no stomach trouble, no hair loss, no pain (except some manageable neuropathy). I just felt weak, dopey, and tired often. I had been stressing about the possible medicinal side effects from what I heard about cancer treatments, only to fly through with none of the effects I tormented myself about. *I learned that a "take it as it comes" attitude is best since I can't predict the future, but I can ruin the present by trying.*

I shifted from some of the active things I enjoyed, like hiking and kayaking, to inactive things that I liked just as much: relaxing in the yard, playing my didgeridoo, watching old movies, and catching up on eating pies. *It's important to remind the sick one of the many enjoyable things they can still do, new ones they can take up, and all there is still to be thankful for.*

PART C. SURVIVAL STATISTICS AND PROGNOSES FUEL A SICK PREJUDICE

1. Why We Want and Expect Statistics

Not knowing what will happen in times of illness can be unsettling. I know I searched for a glimpse of what may happen to me when I was getting cancer so I could be prepared for it. I didn't want to feel out of control and have to respond "on the fly."

Getting some quick online survival statistics or a doctor's prognosis seems to fit the bill perfectly. (A prognosis is typically when a doctor forecasts the likely course of the condition and chances for recovery.) It's a cultural expectation that one of the first questions asked of the doctor is, "What's the prognosis?" It's become an unquestioned part of western medicine to forecast life expectancy and curability. Lots of medical TV shows use the prognosis to heighten drama.

There's an aura of certainty and an almost divine reality around survival statistics. Once we get some idea of "projected survival," we may relax a little, feeling like we have a good idea of what to expect. *Even if it shows a short life expectancy, many believe it's better to feel we know something bad than nothing at all.* Bad news can also confirm the latent, grim feelings we have about sickness, and reinforce the hundreds of high-stress medical drama scenes we've seen on TV.

These statistics come in many forms: Five Year Survival Rates, Survival Curves, Mortality Rates, and Progression Free Survival (for cancer). Do these numbers really help us? I think they can do more harm than good in many cases.

2. How Statistics Add to a Sick Prejudice

Survival statistics can amplify our sick prejudice in at least three ways. First, they focus our thoughts of death and when it is "likely" to happen. Our sick prejudices are already pulling us into sad and morbid feelings. Survival statistics give something seemingly tangible to support those feelings. We are drawn to them like moths to light because it feels natural to be thinking about death when someone gets a serious illness. As we've seen, for 99% of our evolution, death and illness were closely tied together. This is a fundamentally different time now. Death and illness are not nearly as connected as they used to be.

Second, statistics are generalized information about many people who typically have a few similar characteristics, like being a female over age 50 with breast cancer. A sick prejudice results from our generalized experiences and emotions that keep us from thinking about an ill person individually. Survival statistics add to our tendency to rely on generalities about sick people. Generalizations are exactly what keep us from accurately experiencing the unique sick person and situation right in front of us. Often, what we're experiencing instead is something grim and pessimistic. Imagine that you have an illness and your sister who is helping you keeps talking about a girl friend who died from breast cancer after five years, and about some five-year survival statistic she saw about your illness. She is reliving and projecting her experience from a different person onto you. She's not with you. She's somewhere else. We need to be especially personal and present in an illness situation so we can find the particular ways that our loved one will respond best.

Third, survival statistics add to our sick prejudices by starting a sequence of thinking that can worsen our experience as helpers and negatively affect healing outcomes for our sick loved ones. Survival statistics and prognoses are limiting and pessimistic. Whether the average life expectancy is five, ten, or twenty years, who's to say that any one patient isn't going to live longer? Thinking in terms of when death is likely to occur compounds our already morbid and grim tendencies around illness. This can then cripple the healing process and create self-fulfilling prophesies. We start responding in ways regarding our sick loved one that support the assumptions we've made from statistics, rather than understanding them personally. Ultimately, they can start responding in the same way.

3. Problems and Limitations of Survival Statistics

There are several limitations and problems inherent with using statistics and prognoses. One, statistics often come as averages and medians, which can be misleading when used with individual cases because they rarely represent any one person. For example, the median U.S. household income in 2014 is between $50,000 and $54,999 (i.e., $53,657).[16] However, only 4% of households fall into this category. So, you'd be wrong 96% of the time if you guessed the income of $50–55K of someone with no other information other than the average. Yes, if you guessed broader ranges, you'd do increasingly better than 4%, but then your accuracy of their actual income would go down. Similarly, using an average to guess survival is most likely going to be inaccurate.

Two, "survival" type statistics typically include all the

different types of people who had the condition. In the sample, there would be smokers, 80+ year olds, the obese, diabetics, street drug users, people with other serious medical conditions, and many lifestyles and attitudes. Depending on the statistic, they may include people who forgo medical treatment. Our sick friend is different than this hodgepodge sampling, and therefore their results will not be predictable or the same as those of the people used in gathering the statistic.

Three, if our sick loved one is younger than average, the survival statistic wouldn't be a fair measure of how long they have to live. A disproportionately large part of many survival statistics are based on those who are already in their 70s or 80s. Younger patients who use a survival statistic that is based on much older patients are most likely getting an inaccurate outlook of their chances. For example, I was fifty-one when I was diagnosed with cancer. The median age of the statistics for the type of cancer I had was about 70.[17] A study by the American Society of Hematology stated, "In conclusion, patients with myeloma younger than 50 years of age had significantly longer age-adjusted survival both after conventional and high-dose therapy...."[18] So, if I had relied on survival statistics for 70-year-olds, they would have been inaccurate in my case. I would have expected a much shorter life expectancy than would actual happen otherwise. We'll see why this bad in the Exploring How A Sick Prejudice Can Make The Illness Worse section.

Four many survival statistics include all reasons for dying; they're not just counting those dying from the illness in question. This adds more incidents of death and lowers survival time when the average age is in the 70s and 80s. Many chronic health problems occur in elderly people simply because they are more likely to get a serious condition as a part of growing old. Older folks pass on simply from not being strong enough to fight off disease or infections.

Lastly, to get survival statistics, it takes years for the people to die (not to sound callous). By the time the statistic is available, many of the treatments and procedures have been replaced by new ones for which there are no stats yet available.[19] Again, with me, highly effective treatments had come out in the last few years for which there were no statistics for survival or time to relapse. The front-line treatment started moving in just a few years, from stem cell transplants to effective, well tolerated pills and infusions.

When talking to the doctor, it's reasonable *not* to ask for a prognosis or to say you're not interested in one. In my wife's case and mine, we never asked. We didn't need limiting factors. My wife chose to follow all of her doctors' recommendations to the letter. The statistics didn't matter; the best courses of action were advised by her oncologist, neurologist, cardiologist, and surgeon, and she adhered to their directions.

A way to decide whether receiving survival/success statistics is a good choice is to ask: "Are there compelling and immediate actions that would need to be taken based on the data?" In other words, is it worth filling the heads of the sick one and those around them with morbid (and possibly inaccurate) expectations if nothing critical would be done differently? Wills and estates can be done in weeks if needed. There might be little or no choice in the treatment of the illness, anyway, and dwelling on low success rates could reduce the proven beneficial effects of positive expectancy. (Much more on positive expectancy is discussed in Exploring How a Sick Prejudice Can Make the Illness Worse.) *The problem is that once we've seen or heard statistics, we can never go back. They're always in the back of our minds, subduing our enthusiasm, draining our faith, and smothering our human spirit to overcome.*

4. Using Statistics to Help Rather Than Upset Us

All this talk about the issues with survival statistics and getting a prognosis isn't to say they can't be helpful. There are many types of statistics and ways to understand them. Pinpointing ones beneficial to long-term healing and applying them appropriately is the trick, best achieved by open discussions with doctors. Doctors can give us a much more balanced view, rather than making assumptions based on statistics and our own online research.

There are many good uses of survival and treatment/surgery success statistics, such as an elderly patient who doesn't want to go through a painful, difficult medical process if the chances of success are very low (again, thoroughly understanding how those "chances" are derived is crucial). The patient should talk with their doctor and review the appropriate treatment success statistics that are as close as possible to their condition and demographic group. Another example is a patient considering forgoing any conventional treatment or surgery. By getting a prognosis and/or survival data, they could better understand that choice

In reality, it's very difficult to avoid survival and success statistics, even when we want to. Statistics are often embedded in the general information about the disease or illness, which we need in order to query our doctors and make good choices. It takes self-discipline to keep statistics' limitations in mind and to forbid them from influencing our thoughts. A good doctor is the best choice over online statistics and research because they can evaluate the person's unique condition and medical history, is up-to-date on medical trials, and considers all this within a full treatment plan.

CHAPTER II. EXPLORING HOW A SICK PREJUDICE CAN MAKE THE ILLNESS WORSE

A sick prejudice sits squarely between the help and relationships that chronically ill people need, and those who can give it to them (i.e., us). The level of caring and compassion we show, the quality of interactions we have, and our love and friendship for a sick person can make a real life-or-death difference in their recovery.

A large analysis of 148 related studies involving over 308,000 participants, "Social Relationships and Mortality Risk: A Meta-analytic Review,"[20] concluded, in part, that "people with stronger social relationships had a 50% increased likelihood of survival than those with weaker social relationships."

Further, "These findings indicate that the influence of social relationships on the risk of death is comparable with well-established risk factors for mortality such as smoking and alcohol consumption and exceed the influence of other risk factors such as physical inactivity and obesity."[21]

Our mishmash of fears, assumptions, and stereotypes about someone sick can create at least two large problems. First, they can push us away from the sick one and cause us to avoid them.

As we've seen, this steals a critical healing mechanism from them and an enriching opportunity for us. Second, even when we do decide to get more involved, a sick prejudice can create an unhealthy environment and undermine healing for someone ill. We can impress our own pessimistic, scared, and dire outlook of the situation onto the sick one.

How might this happen? Through the power of negative expectancy. A way to understand this can be seen through the placebo and nocebo effects (yes, it's really called the "nocebo"). Let's look in some detail at how they work and how they can help explain the influence friends and family have on someone ill.

PART A. THE PLACEBO EFFECT

Everyone is generally familiar with the placebo effect. Here is a medical definition from a MedicineNet.com article: "Placebo effect: Also called the Placebo response. A remarkable phenomenon in which a Placebo—a fake treatment, an inactive substance like sugar, distilled water, or saline solution—can sometimes improve a patient's condition simply because the person has the expectation that it will be helpful. Expectation plays a potent role in the Placebo effect. The more a person believes they are going to benefit from a treatment, the more likely it is that they will experience a benefit."[22] What patients expect can and does affect them, usually regarding symptoms of pain, depression, anxiety, fatigue, and certain emotionally sensitive conditions.[23] It's like the role encouragement plays in accomplishing goals in our everyday lives. We use it with our work teams, children, and ourselves.

In a WebMD article called "What Is the Placebo Effect," we see how easily we can respond to expectations: "For instance, in one study, people were given a Placebo and told it was a stimulant. After taking the pill, their pulse rate sped up, their blood pressure increased, and their reaction speeds improved. When people were given the same pill and told it was to help them get to sleep they experienced the opposite effects."[24]

In another article called "Placebo Effects in Medicine," by Ted J. Kaptchuk and Franklin G. Miller, PhD., published in *The New England Journal of Medicine*, it says "Research suggests that distinct neurobiologic mechanisms are activated. Empathic health care creates a cognitive-affective-sensory orientation, tapping into conscious and nonconscious mechanisms that can predispose patients toward reduced symptom severity and lessened reactivity to underlying pathophysiology. Or to borrow terms from the behavioral social sciences, healing interactions 'frame,' 'anchor,' or 'nudge' patients toward shifts in their perceptions of their symptoms and illness, making them less disturbed or perturbed."[25]

As you may know, one of the most important elements in drug trials has been controlling for the placebo effect. That's because if patients can improve themselves, then the drug doesn't add anything. The placebo effect is so sensitive that not only are the patients not told who gets the medicine and who gets the "sugar pills," but the doctors and nurses aren't told, either, so that no subtle cues can be transmitted (i.e., "double blind").[26] This is important to us, because it speaks to how just a hint of expectation by someone can sway results, let alone how influential our visible fears and morbid expectations can be.

PART B. THE NOCEBO EFFECT

The frightening prospect that could be influenced by a sick prejudice is the opposite of the placebo. The nocebo effect occurs
when people make themselves feel worse by believing they took
something or that some condition is making them sick, when
there actually isn't something making them sick. Dr. Lissa
Rankin's article, "The Nocebo Effect: Negative thoughts can harm
your health," states: "But the Placebo effect has a shadow side.
The same mind-body power that can heal you can also harm you.
When patients in double-blinded clinical trials are warned about
the side effects they may experience if they're given the real drug,
approximately 25% experience sometimes severe side effects,
even when they're only taking sugar pills. Those treated with
nothing more than Placebos often report fatigue, vomiting,
muscle weakness, colds, ringing in the ears, taste
disturbances, memory disturbances, and other symptoms that
shouldn't result from a sugar pill."[27] Further, negative emotions
and doubt can potentially make people feel worse as seen in a
study abstract, "Nocebo—The Opposite of Placebo." It's
concluded that, "Nocebo-stimuli, such as anxiety, fear, mistrust
and doubt, may reduce a Placebo-effect; it may induce negative

side-effects in Placebo-treatment; it may produce new aversive symptoms; and it may reverse symptoms from positive ones to negative ones (e.g. revert an analgesic response to hyperalgesia)."[28] These nocebo stimuli are also some of the same stimuli of a sick prejudice (i.e., fear, anxiety, and mistrust of getting involved).

PART C. DOCTORS' INTERACTION STYLE CAN HINDER OR HELP

The way in which doctors and nurses interact with patients can also impact their response. Cara Feinberg's 2013 *Harvard Magazine* article, "The Placebo Phenomenon: An ingenious researcher (i.e., Ted J. Kaptchuk) finds the real ingredients of 'fake' medicine," summarizes Ted Kaptchuk: "It's valuable insight for any caregiver: patients' perceptions matter, and the ways physicians frame perceptions can have significant effects on their patients' health."[29] In a study by Massachusetts General Hospital, it was found that the relationship doctors have with patients can affect patient results. Lead author John M. Kelley, PhD, said: "Our results show that the beneficial effects of a good patient-clinician relationship on health care outcomes are of similar magnitude to many well-established medical treatments."[30]

It doesn't seem too much of a stretch for us as helpers to leverage similar positive effects as the "good patient-clinician relationship." When we consider that we can spend much more time with our sick friend than they spend with doctors, and that the level of trust and bonding we have with them from years of being together can be much deeper, our influence on their expectations could be pivotal. Imagine having a serious condition and your good friend is steadfastly confident that you will get better. Everything they do shows they assume that. Conversely, imagine them as worried, fear in their eyes and constantly thinking about losing you and how terrible that would be. I always knew with my condition that something would work. There were some dark times when I would gobble up the worst thoughts like a cruddy chocolate raspberry cake at a banquet. Almost all the time though, I pushed the cruddy cake of despair away. (More primary research of the effects of certain home and care-giver conditions on healing outcomes is needed.)

PART D. OUR INTERACTION STYLE AS HELPERS CAN HINDER OR HELP

What does all this placebo and nocebo stuff mean to us? Clearly, sick people can be affected by what they believe is going to happen to them as a result of the power of positive and negative expectation. The emotional "climate" and interactions patients have can influence outcomes. The long-term effect of reducing symptoms of pain, fatigue, and depression by invoking placebo and eliminating nocebo type responses could improve eating, sleeping, activity, and general strength. These in turn can be beneficial to overall healing outcomes by enabling more tolerance to treatments and surgeries, if nothing else.

What's being suggested here is that the frequent looks and voices of fear, tragedy, and resignation from trusted loved ones is perhaps as powerful and condemning to someone sick as believing a fake treatment is going to cause harmful side-effects. Our sick loved one may be scared and thinking solemn, grave thoughts already. If we as helpers have similar thoughts and commiserate with them, it confirms their worries that this is a dreadful situation. Further, as we've seen, it can start a cycle of unfortunate self-fulfilling prophesies.

We can be a decisive part of their healing process. We've all heard the many cases of patients ignoring how much time doctors have said they have and going on to live much longer or even recovering fully. We need to work through our sick prejudices and give our loved one the emotional support to beat "the odds."

It starts with what we often consider the obligatory response to hearing someone is diagnosed with a major health problem: *"Oh my God! That's terrible! I'm so sorry." In a few seconds, we've communicated shock, fright, tragedy, and sadness. As friends and family, we've solidified our expectation that the sick one is in for a dreadful time and has one foot in the grave.* It's understandable that we say this. We don't want to seem like we're uncaring, and we assume that the sick one probably feels like a tragedy has happened to them. The fact is, we don't know what will happen in the months and years to come. We do know now that positive expectancy and encouragement are a lot better than framing the situation in ominous, foreboding terms.

I remember a defining moment when I was telling some co-workers that I had cancer. One of them had a reaction like above. The first thing he said was: "What's the prognosis"? This is like asking, "How long do you have to live?" I said, "I didn't ask for a prognosis." His jaw dropped and he looked noticeably disappointed, as though I neglected a key part of getting a serious illness. Then, I explained how I'm different from the statistics and that I planned to just go through the process and do well (which I did). The other co-worker understood this and calmly nodded. I think some people expect to be a part of that emotional prognosis scene in a TV medical drama, and then give others the somber news about how long the person has to live. I hope my news of the illness was relayed more like: "Joe has cancer, is feeling pretty good, is just taking it as it comes and thinks everything is going to work out well."

When I was in treatment, I didn't want people worrying about me. I viewed that as negative, fear-based energy that focused on bad things possibly happening. I didn't want them praying that certain "bad" things didn't happen either. I wanted them to believe (and pray) that things would go well. I wanted them to have faith that it would work out. Fortunately, they did, and I did my part to get well. Let's continually hold thoughts that our sick friend is strong and in a transitional state between healthy periods. We'll look for the good in their journey. It was as simple for my wife and me as having calmness, faith, and persistence in good outcomes. In Figure 2, we can see the possible chain of events starting from what we believe and ending with the outcomes experienced.

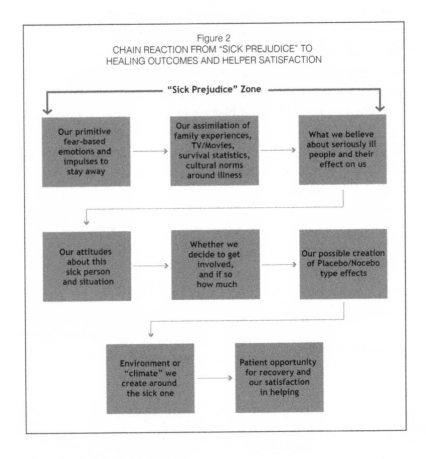

Figure 2
CHAIN REACTION FROM "SICK PREJUDICE" TO
HEALING OUTCOMES AND HELPER SATISFACTION

MARY MORRISSEY, best-selling author and president of Life-SOULutions, found miraculous results from resolutely holding on to the simple fact that, of all the possible outcomes, there is at least one where the sick person (or ourselves) are healed and cured. We can believe firmly in that outcome.[31] There are a lot of inspiring sources and stories that reinforce healing and wellness. Know that even if our sick loved one isn't confident, they can effectively "borrow" our confidence.[32] They trust us. Even if they are doubtful from an intellectual standpoint, their hopeful emotions gleaned from our confidence can give them placebo-type effects.[33] If limiting information has already been heard, gently and continually move their focus to living, wellness, and the possible outcome of getting better. Talk about future plans, so they feel the temporary nature of their illness. If it is their time to go, it will become apparent, and no statistic is needed to tell us that. Even then, having faith that their passing/transition will be filled with love and joy for all the good times is a gift for everyone.

CHAPTER III. SICK PREJUDICE AVOIDANCE TACTICS THAT KEEP US FROM HELPING

PART A. THE NINE SIDELINE EXCUSES AND CONCERNS

When feelings of a sick prejudice are present, we look for excuses and reasons to justify what we want—to avoid the sick person and situation as much as we reasonably can. The excuses we tell ourselves make very good sense to us and might contain some truth. The problem is that we are in a biased state of mind and seeing things in a way that supports the bias. We can as easily choose to believe we know little about this sickness situation, what it will be like to provide support, and that we'll take it as it comes. These nine excuses in particular can keep us on the sidelines instead of with our sick friend or loved one.

I. "There is nothing I can do or there must be someone else who can help."

In the back of our minds, we might think, "There's nothing I can really do. It's just going to be hard for them." This is an avoidance excuse. With little effort, there's usually a lot we can do to make life easier for them and more fulfilling for us. Start with something shorter like a few hours or a single chore once a week. What the right amount is will be much clearer by "dipping a toe in" rather than speculating about how it will work. Even short, occasional assistance can mean a lot to the sick person and importantly shows them that someone cares. This, in turn, can translate into self-worth at a time when it is needed most.

An easy "out" is to tell ourselves there must be other people or family (if we're friends) who can step in besides us. For the most part, it's safe to assume, until shown otherwise, that sick folks or those helping them can always use some support. That doesn't mean being around the house every day, but being available and willing to do some things. (Please see the Helping section for more ideas on how to help in manageable ways that work for all parties.)

2. "Now that I think about it, I'm not really that close with the person."

We may start questioning how close our relationship really is with the sick one—which means we're in sick prejudice territory. If we believe we're not really that close, then our sense of duty or obligation is reduced. As it turns out, we don't have to have a close relationship to support those who are ill. In fact, it's often easier for someone less intimate to assist—there's no strained history or expectations. One relative who helped my daughter and me in the crucial months after my wife died was actually not directly related to either of us. Not having a close relationship to start with is a nice opportunity to find new meaning in a time of needing and giving.

"I'll just offer to help…if anything is ever needed." This statement can translate into, "I don't really want to help much, if at all. You're going to have to just get through it for a while, and I'm going now." It is rarely easy for people to ask for help, so don't place the burden back on the sick person. Time and energy are limited for the sick, so they probably don't have the wherewithal to pull together a list of chores and call people.

If we really want them to call and are just being polite, there are more concrete approaches. Call them. When we're at their house visiting, we can look around and see what needs doing. Are there dishes in the sink? Is the refrigerator empty? Does the dog need walking? Do the floors need vacuuming or mopping? Do the kids need an outing? We can just do it then if appropriate, or give them a day and time when we can.

3. "It's their fault they're sick from always doing..."

We may blame the sick one for their illness. It's easy and convenient for us to stand in judgment of how they lived and find reasons they may have caused it.

When there's an attitude of "They deserve what they get," that lets us off the hook. A research study called "Perceptions of Health and Illness" stated: "Research has shown that people will avoid cancer patients if they view the patient as contributing to the disease."[34]

The findings probably apply to other illnesses as well and represent a general attitude. A person could ask, "What if their illness could've been caused by something they did, like smoking cigarettes their whole life? Are we supposed to spend our time helping them?" The short answer is, "Yes." It doesn't matter why they're sick, just that they need some care.

We can't fully understand why people do the things they do, what influences they had growing up, or why things happen to some and not others. If folks need support, we pitch in and help. It's much easier than our sick prejudices lead us to believe.

4. "I'm getting irritated that they..."

We may feel irritated by many different things—their complaining, their messy house, how they talk to us or other people in their family. There's no limit to the things we can let get on our nerves. *The "emotional sunburn factor" mentioned earlier can get red and sensitive as we spend time helping. Any sick prejudice we have is looking for a way out of the situation. If it can't find it in other ways, it will try being irritated and ticked off.*

This certainly isn't to say that what we're feeling is all a perception on our part. Sick people are not always easy to be around or on their best behavior. It's natural for them to be irritable, rude, and impolite at times. Add medications and treatments on top of illness, and their moods are affected even more. If they're in pain, they may be especially prone to irritability. Irritability when sick is normal, widespread, and is even documented in other species.[35] They may not be particularly thankful.

So, there are two things happening here. One, our emotions as helpers can be heightened, making us feel hypersensitive and impatient with the situation. Two, the sick one is being emotionally bounced around, causing them to behave poorly and unlike themselves. This is all happening in a home environment that has probably become messier and lower functioning. Sickness breaks the usual living processes.

Sometimes when we had family visiting us, they clearly resented doing the laundry and chores. It made everything worse. We felt like we had to tiptoe around them so they would not get upset. We became more and more reluctant to ask them to come out and help because the friction was a big cost and drain and not much help. In one case, the helper appeared visibly irritated and impatient and did poor work, with the result of us resolving not to ask them to come out again unless it was the direst of situations.

How we react to these changes in ourselves, the sick one, and the environment is the key. We need to expect that negative interactions will happen at times. Even when we are not thanked, we can know that we accomplished useful things. We can't let things irritate us to a point where we limit the care we give to those in need. We just let our sick loved one's emotions come and go and not take things personally. When we feel ourselves getting irritated, we step away, take a walk, breathe, and talk to the sick one about what's happening as appropriate. Our expectations of the sick one and how things get done need to change so that we are accepting, forgiving, and understanding. As long as schedules are being kept for meals, medicines, bathroom needs, and doctor appointments, things are going all right. Our expectations are reduced, and we're just looking at getting by day-to-day.

5. "I don't like being around sick people, in their homes, or going to hospitals."

This is not so much an excuse as a reality for some who might have repulsion of sickness, hospitals, sickness situations, and of how the patient looks and smells. They might experience claustrophobia cooped up in a bedroom or hospital room. Perhaps their sick prejudices and feelings about illness are not something they can use their will to overcome. I occasionally had tinges of these feelings at times when I was young, and I've heard others talk about it. A good solution is to help the helpers of the sick person. Do things to support those who are in direct contact with the sick one. Whatever aid can be given allows them to spend more time and energy where needed and wanted. Consider also that perhaps like reducing other fears (swimming, public speaking, pulling onto freeways, etc.), practice could lessen these feelings; try spending short durations with the sick person or at the hospital (and then leave with great relief and a skip in your step, which is okay).

6. "It seems like they're milking this for all it's worth."

It can seem like the sick person is exaggerating their symptoms for attention. This belief may stem from both actual behaviors by the sick one and heightened emotions from a sick prejudice in the helper. There are deep, innate sickness behaviors (i.e., a "sick role") that humans have so that others will know we are sick and can come to our aid.[36] Expect some needy, "wimpy" behavior at times, as a sick child would have. Also, the overall situation may be more difficult than friends and family understand; if they did, perhaps they would be whiny too. The benefit of the doubt needs to be with the sick one.

When I was first being diagnosed with multiple myeloma (a blood cancer), I needed some people to feel sorry for me at times and give me some special attention. My wife was always good with that. I'd go through a kind of stunned "Woe is me" attitude for a few hours or days. Then I was onto the next emotion until I had tried them all out. I pretty much settled back to where I was before the diagnosis.

We might also blame the sick one for our feelings of guilt about not getting involved more. A little voice in us may say, "Are all these complaints of theirs so I will be 'guilted' into helping more?" Feeling guilty is normal, but no one can make us feel guilty; we do it to ourselves. How we deal with guilt is what matters. These feelings are a cue for us to stop and look at how we are thinking about the situation. It's important we don't feel like we're being pulled into doing something out of guilt or desperation. That leads to resentment, which taints the healing environment. We can reevaluate the kind and amount of support we are giving to ensure it is satisfactory to us long-term. We may, in fact, be happier assisting with more, leaving no doubt in our minds that we put in a solid effort. If we let it build, though, it can hurt them and us.

7. "I don't want to interfere or butt-in."

This excuse can be made out of seeming consideration for the sick one and their family, but the person with this excuse only makes it if they haven't or aren't planning to ask the sick one about their needs. If they had asked to help in earnest, they would know if it was a bother. If a person wants to be of service, they should make it clearly known and offer unsolicited help. (Please see further discussion in the Helping section.)

8. "Will I feel so bad for them I'll end up offering to do more than I'm comfortable doing?"

Thinking about helping an ill friend or loved one over a longer term can trigger concerns about giving more to the situation than we want. I know I've thought this way. "I'm not sure how much I really want to know." This reaction is probably the most important, thorny side of sick prejudice. Fear of something bad happening to us by getting involved with a sick person is a core reason for not wanting to learn more so that we aren't drawn too close to them. We're limiting what we can know about this situation based on what we *think* we will hear and feel. We're assuming a chronic illness situation is going to be bad and that it's best to not get involved. So, we may avoid the whole situation before we even know what's really needed and how it feels.

We can manage our involvement, which feels good. We don't need to fear that the situation will overwhelm us. We can learn to say, "I won't be able to do that at this point, but I could do _____ instead." It's strengthening to effectively and compassionately set our boundaries. It felt good to know that I could manage the situation. Whatever level of support we choose, we'll have lots of time to adjust as we go. Just saying some kind words is a great way to start and to feel a sense of satisfaction.

I found that the importance of a sick person's need and my self-satisfaction always balanced out—the greater their need, the greater my satisfaction in helping. I never felt used or unappreciated. As Gordon B. Hinckley said, "One of the great ironies of life is this: He or she who serves almost always benefits more than he or she who is served."[37] There are many quotes like these. The problem is that no matter how much sense these kinds of quotes make to us intellectually, our deep-seated emotions and sick prejudices can override them. That's why we just need to jump in, start doing things to help, and experience how it feels. Over time, then, our experiences outweigh our assumptions and inherited emotions, tipping the scales in favor of everyone involved.

9. "I'm afraid I'll be overwhelmed by their problems."

We may also worry that the sick person will say things that will be too overwhelming and troubling for us, and we don't know if we can deal with those feelings. Occasionally I would feel unequipped to deal with the problems mentioned. My father had Parkinson's. In the later stages, he suffered greatly, and there were incredibly difficult situations to face. It should be expected that we aren't immediately going to know how to think about things we haven't had to face before. For me, it took some experimentation. I found that the problems I heard about always resolved in the days and weeks to follow as I let go of my illness assumptions, found calmness, and simply accepted the illness situation as it was.

For some folks, hearing the "gory details" of the person's illness is a big, uncomfortable obstacle. They just don't want to do it. That's okay too, and probably the sick one will sense that, and the conversations will stay on lighter subjects. Either way—understanding their problems deeply, or not—it will feel good to be with the person before it's too late to make a difference.

PART B. KNOWING WE'RE RESPONDING FROM THE PAST

It's important we understand that the causes of our sick prejudice —primitive responses, family influences, prior experiences with illness, survival statistics, and stories we've heard—are all from the past. This means we're feeling and responding to things that don't exist anymore. Our assumptions and stereotypes not only have all the flaws mentioned above, but they are no longer relevant. Sickness evokes seemingly dire circumstances, creating even more temptation to use whatever limited experiences we can dredge up from the past.

The idea then is to constantly keep ourselves in the present moment, especially when having conversations with the sick one about their illness. Staying present keeps us focused on the person we're tending to rather than some past ill loved one or implanted feeling. Just being aware when we reflect on an experience or something outside of this situation can enable us to stop and look at the facts about our sick friend. We need to be with just our sick loved one and take it moment-to-moment. Being open in this way and maintaining faith in positive outcomes allows good things for everyone to work their way in. Otherwise, we constrain what can happen by expectations taken from some-where else.

CHAPTER IV. MANAGING A SICK PREJUDICE AND ENABLING A HEALING ENVIRONMENT

PART A. UNDERSTANDING AND TREATING THE SICK PERSON AS AN INDIVIDUAL

Learning about the sick one personally is at the core of eliminating our sick prejudice. By definition, we are not prejudiced or using stereotypes when we think of someone as an individual and not as part of some group we're generalizing about. Just as we can learn to respect and work with people from different backgrounds, ideologies, and lifestyles when we get to know them as an individual, so too can we feel good about aiding a sick person when we get to know them and their situation better. We can let go of the past, of statistics, TV dramas, or primitive sickness emotions, when we understand someone personally. We see just the issues and opportunities with this one person today.

We simply need to ask them how it's going. They may talk superficially at first, so they don't feel like they're complaining or "scaring us off" by jumping into serious issues too soon. Just keep listening and gently probing. At times, our loved one can naturally be feeling overwhelmed and get carried into exaggeration and negative scenarios when they talk. Just being heard can be therapeutic for them, and listening qualifies for help on our part.

Please keep in mind that each of us has unique feelings about having a life-threatening illness. Realizing this uniqueness is a large part of combatting sick prejudice and seeing them as our loved one, not as their illness or another ill person we know. Some common questions and concerns that sick folks can have are listed below.

1. Will I be in pain?
2. Will I get better?
3. How will I do everything while being sick?
4. What will happen to my job?
5. What will happen to my quality of life?
6. How do I take care of my family and home?
7. How will my loved ones be affected?
8. How bad will I feel during treatment and/or surgeries?
9. What will the recovery be like and how long will it take?

The answers to most of their questions and ours will be played out gradually. I found that time, reassurance, and a few good facts are more important than any future speculation. As Eckhart Tolle said in his book, *The Power of Now*, "You can always cope with the present moment, but you cannot cope with something that is only a mind projection - you cannot cope with the future."[38] I became aware of future thinking that my wife and I would easily slip into, and particularly the words "What if...?" "What if" scenarios, when combined with the heightened emotions of sickness, can create almost paranoid thinking. I got used to saying, "Let's wait and see what happens."

Further probing about how your loved one or friend feels might reveal deeper, almost remorseful emotions. They may feel disappointed in themselves, have low self-esteem, and even feel shame because they can do so little and need so much. They may wonder if they did something terribly wrong in their lives, such as "angered the Gods," or that karma is at work.[39] They may feel guilt for causing problems. They may grieve for the life they had, similar to losing a loved one. They may be indulging in fatalistic thinking by looking at statistics and getting prognoses. These feelings can shift a person into a sad and resigned state of being. We need to gently keep moving them into this moment, or if "now" is painful, encouraging them about a healed, enjoyable future.

Chronic sickness can be an incredibly lonely time, especially those suffering from the effects of a sick prejudice or someone completely without family and friends. Shannon L. Alder said, "One of the most important things you can do on earth is to let people know they are not alone."[40] This is why even those quick visits and little gestures can make a difference.

PART B. REALIZING THE SICK ONE HAS SICK PREJUDICES, TOO

Sick folks are likely distressed by the same sickness stereotypes, assumptions, fears, and errors in thinking that everyone else is. Worse, it's all intensified by treatments, surgeries, and the instability of drug-induced emotions. Not surprisingly, they can start thinking that people want to avoid them and stay away from the situation. They don't want to be an imposition, may fear hurting a relationship, or might think people are just being polite when they offer to help. *They can even start pushing people and assistance away, believing that's what should happen to sick people: they should be abandoned.*

Rattling around in the back of their minds (and ours) may be the old saying, "If you don't have your health, you don't have anything." The saying is well intentioned, but the fact is it's not true. First, the ill person may be healthy except for the one large problem (e.g., cancer, heart, etc.) and the complications it may cause. They need to be careful not to think they've "lost all their health," because of one thing, albeit a big thing. Fix the one thing, and they can be back to the way they were. Second, they can still have a lot of enjoyable things in their life—friends, favorite shows, family, pets, interests, art, music, hobbies, memories, nature—and the same dreams we all share.

In some cases, the sick one or their family members will be in denial that something substantial has happened in their life. Perhaps their primitive fears and assumptions about sickness are too overwhelming to face. How people react may be influenced by the emotional stages of a chronic illness they are experiencing.* The stages can include feelings of Crisis, Denial, Anger, Isolation, Reconstruction, and Acceptance. I found the stages weren't optional and happened sequentially over time. I needed to pass through one to get to the next. *My innate fears and a lifetime of assumptions about illness (i.e., my sick prejudice) threaded their way through these stages, holding me back from moving through them as easily as I would have otherwise.* The Crisis stage was hard for me with my already nervous disposition. The Isolation stage was long and overlapped with other stages. It was the stage that prompted the idea for this book.

A serious illness is an experiential process that patients, their families, and even friends can move through over time. It's similar to the grieving process when a loved one passes away. It's vitally important that everyone involved in a newly diagnosed chronic illness realize that they will feel differently in the long run than they do in the first couple of months.

PART C. SPECIAL FOCUS—LIVING WITH ILLNESS IN A MARRIAGE OR LOVING PARTNERSHIP

1. Possible Effects and Changes

Sickness can be especially hard on spouses and significant others. Living together not only can raise sensitivity to the "sunburn factor" (i.e., getting irritable by otherwise normal requests and preferences), but can intensify our primitive responses, memories of past experiences, and other sick prejudice symptoms. It's important not to underestimate the toll and changes a serious illness can have on a marriage.

Basic reasons that the couple came into the relationship can change, at least temporarily. Maybe the sick one was an active, outdoor, energetic person. Now they're lethargic and sullen. They can naturally be needier, uncomfortable, and in pain. The sick one can be moody and look and smell different.

In general, the healthy partner may be doing more of the chores, participating in fewer activities, getting less exercise, missing vacations, having little or no sex, cooking more, and tending to emotional children. Compounding things further, it can feel like it makes matters worse to talk about some of these things with the sick partner. These life changes can be the biggest things going on in the well partner's life. Now more than ever they need their closest confidant to talk to about all of this, but there can be the legitimate concern that talking to their sick loved one could make them feel worse than they already do.

A sudden illness in a marriage or for those living together can be traumatic and demanding, unlike with a friend or other loved one living elsewhere. When my wife got sick, it was life altering. A lot changed. It was a little like the birth of a child in that our lifestyle completely changed from one day to the next, except without the cuteness. There were new chores, errands, sleepless nights, and frequent care the sickness required. The medications, doctor appointments, pain, and limitations were with us throughout every day for twelve years.

The couple's social and extended family life will likely change a lot. When a sick prejudice kicks in, some friends and family will no longer be around like they used to. Even if they are around, there can start to be little in common with friends who don't have a major illness, with not much else for the sick couple to talk about. It can be too much trouble to entertain at home. Both partners can end up withdrawing from social situations. This was part of the journey for my wife and me. Over time, it can become isolating as friends dwindle away from lack of socializing and possibly sick prejudices. It's worrisome to lose connection, in case help is suddenly needed. It takes a conscious effort to keep communication open and visits regular with friends and family.

If the illness goes on for years, the well partner's physical and emotional health can deteriorate, and they can get illnesses of their own. Ultimately, this then affects our sick loved one as well. Taking care of ourselves as helpers is vitally important with a live-in relationship. It's best in the long-term for us to maintain our active lives, even if our partner can't participate. Continuing our activities, hobbies, sports, and keeping up with friends is essential.

2. Pitfalls in the Diagnosis Stage

Probably the most crucial time to be keenly aware of our sick prejudice tendencies is during the first weeks of a serious illness. We can be an emotional mess if we don't realize they are there, or we can be a confident and calm presence when we do. When my wife first became ill on that camping trip in mid-2002, I started calling hospitals and connecting with all family and friends to find a suitable place for her to get diagnosed. In that process, I wanted to be diligent and knowledgeable. I spent dozens of hours researching her illnesses in the days that she was being diagnosed (and misdiagnosed). Unfortunately, most of the research and statistics kept me in a frantic state of mind, particularly since I was already emotionally amped-up on sick prejudices.

As can be the case during the diagnosis stage, doctors would give their best guesses as to what the problem was, which kept me bouncing from disease to disease online, trying to keep ahead of it all. What was thought to be lung cancer turned out to be thymoma—a very big difference. What appeared on an MRI to be a metastasized brain tumor needing skull surgery was determined by a newer MRI at a top hospital to be an old calcium deposit requiring no treatment. She sometimes said, "I'd have to have a hole in my head to do...." Fortunately, testing continued at a national hospital, and she never had to have that hole in her head.

I learned several crucial lessons during this time. First, get multiple opinions and a diagnosis from a doctor who commonly works with the particular illness, preferably at a top medical institution. This may take time and several interviews with doctors. Second, find someone you like, trust, and can talk to easily. My wife ended up with a perfect doctor (i.e., close connection and highly competent). Ten years later, when I became ill, I found an easygoing doctor with a wise view of the research and the patience to discuss my detailed questions. Third, the diagnosis process may "bounce around" before settling in on the final conclusion. It's important to question the reasoning behind the diagnosis until you feel comfortable and to keep a light, wait-and-see attitude along the way. *Fourth, stay vigilant of everyone involved for the false sense of urgency, somber outlook, and subtle life-or-death desperation of a sick prejudice.*

We need to have faith in the unique healing abilities of our loved one (or ourselves) and the effectiveness of treatment plans. *Then, once a plan is decided, let the doctors do their jobs, and the medicines work their miracles, and keep the sick one focused on other areas of their lives (eating well, exercise/activity, spirituality/church, hobbies/interests, etc.).*

3. Managing and Getting Along

When we're married, or living with the sick person, we especially need to communicate a lot. They will most likely be wondering about the same things as we are and possibly assuming the worst. We can keep it lighter, optimistic, and filled with love. I found it was easier to have more frequent, brief conversations as the thoughts arose. Something might pop out during dinner, or while watching TV, or just before bed. We needed to talk at many different times and in many places to find a balanced perspective. Each couple can be different. It may be better to discuss it all at once and be done with it for some couples, rather having it around all the time. It will be important to be sensitive to their cues and yours.

At one of our early doctor appointments, I expressed my feelings of being overwhelmed. I felt like I was cramming for a final exam with no opportunity for failure. The doctor said something like, "Oh, that's right, you're still quite new to all of this and haven't had time to learn the new job." Caring for an ill loved one is like any new job or change. It's an adjustment at first and with time becomes more comfortable and routine.

When my wife was sick, I continued to kayak, hike, and even occasionally go on a vacation (she didn't mind getting rid of me for a little while!). Don't let family vacations and outings dwindle away completely. They can be shorter, easier, and less often. Don't be afraid to make plans. Schedule them on a calendar. They can always be pushed back or reduced if needed. There are usually opportunities for having some fun if you look. My wife and I needed to make regularly scheduled trips to UCLA. While there, we'd go to the beaches, see sights, eat out, kick back in the hotel room, and make a vacation out of the trips.

It's essential to take good care of our health when our partner is very ill. Not only can we take better care of them if we are feeling well, but our sustained good energy from a wholesome lifestyle pulls up the enthusiasm of our sick one. I realized this early on and improved my eating, kept exercising, took it easier at work, got more sleep, and pursued spirituality. Additionally, there may not be anyone available or willing to look after us or our sick partner if we get health problems.

The well partner's needs will likely get lost in the sick partner's major health issues at some point. They can feel their needs are not being met or are unseen with all the attention on the sick one. We need to catch this before we start feeling trapped, sullen, or angry. Otherwise, over time, this can lead to depressed feelings and vicious cycles that affect everyone around us.

Even with our best efforts of caring for ourselves, we can gradually get run down over time. It can happen easier when we're the type that's overly caring and empathetic, as I was. I had a subconscious feeling that the family was in a low-level, constant crisis. That can wear anybody down over the years, especially those who are more sensitive. When signs of wear start appearing, we must find ways to understand them and get support. To start, taking some time off, reevaluating our approach, and talking with friends and family can provide needed perspective. *We need to be completely honest about the impact our caregiving is having on us. Our friends and family need to be completely open to that impact, even if it means they may have to step in and do more.* This can get tricky with a sick prejudice looming in the background.

A higher level of care may be needed for the sick partner. That's a very difficult conclusion to come to, but if it isn't made when needed, we can end up with two sick people needing care. Other people and resources then must be pulled in. We will often think that without our current level of involvement, the sick person will not be cared for enough. Whether it is true or not that they will be cared for like we would do, they usually can be cared for adequately.

All these issues certainly don't have to add up to an unsatisfactory relationship or loss of love. *In fact, sickness can make the relationship grow stronger and the love deeper.* In our relationship, there was a level of love that I think would've been impossible to experience without great challenges. I developed more compassion and understanding for people going through hardship than I ever could have otherwise. That will be a gift I carry with me for the rest of my life.

I'm sure that a good marriage can not only survive, but thrive in the face of illness because what's most important in life is each other. Start by letting go of expectations and how things used to be. Also, don't hesitate to ask others for help if you want it. It lets people know it's needed and can shake them out of some of their sick prejudice if they're having some conflict due to that.

As caregivers, being aware of our internal fear-based triggers is a big part of the battle of treating our own sick prejudice and making the most of the circumstances. Increasing our awareness of our feelings and the choices we make, and testing them for truth, improves matters substantially. Trying different ways of supporting the sick one and getting real information rather than speculating about what will happen is a valuable way to navigate the care we give and the relationship we have.

It's important to frequently talk about how we feel. We can talk to friends, relatives, counselors, support groups, spouses, online chat groups, meet-up groups, barbers, and hair stylists. Hearing what others have experienced reassures us that we are not alone and can do it. Support groups meet in most cities. Processing about the illness can't be done all in our heads; talking is essential. Support groups for caregivers can give us a new perspective and make us feel less alone.

Reading stories by other people going through similar circumstances is both valuable and comforting. Stories about people's struggles and how people have made illness a growth time in their lives were some of the best stories I've ever read. They gave me strength I didn't know I had. I found them through books, articles, and online sources. Remember not to use this tool for answers or prognoses, but rather as inspiration for how to thrive in difficult times.

4. Family Support

There are many sides to family support, or the lack thereof. It's difficult and filled with "defining moments" and decisions. There are varying needs by a sick person for family, from not being able to get by without them, to having no need for them at all. In my wife's case, we didn't need day-to-day help with chores or errands for about eight of the twelve years. Her family was out of state (I didn't have any family then). They were content to call weekly, and my wife would talk and give them a mild version that was digestible for their tolerances.

There was family support for emergencies like taking my wife to the ER, and for surgeries when I simply couldn't be in several places at once: work, home with kids, and at the hospital. A member of my wife's family would come out in those instances and stay until we were basically self-sufficient again.

We were very grateful for that. Coming out for emergencies and returning to their own lives afterward is a reasonable thing. During the last few of the twelve years, we were sent some money for housekeeping and yard work, also a helpful and very appreciated gesture.

The problem was there was no support for the long-term decline in opportunity over almost twelve years: reduced career growth, spent financial savings, emotional tolls, lost life experiences, and the partner's health (i.e., mine!).

The long march down can go uncovered. For that, family is needed in the area to spread the responsibility so that more than just the married couple bears it all.

Relocating can obviously have a number of obstacles for family thinking of moving near their sick one: loss of current friends and work contacts, attachment to an area, and being put into what can be perceived as a burdensome support position.

Distance forces less involvement and protects the current lifestyle. Unfortunately, not being there for a beloved family member during their hardest times can be a loss greater than keeping the status quo elsewhere. For extended family, it seems safe to assume that it will feel good to be close to your sick loved one and that it will work out for the best somehow.

There will be tough choices with no "right" answers. Be guided by how you would like things to be when your time comes to need help.

PART D. THE GREAT EIGHT PAIN RELIEVERS FOR A SICK PREJUDICE

Below is a quick "prescription" for managing a sick prejudice. It summarizes the key take-aways of this book. Read it daily when you hear of a friend or family member getting a serious illness, or if know of someone now.

The Great Eight Pain Relievers For A Sick Prejudice

Dosage: Read once daily for the first month and as needed thereafter to maintain a sense of calm, purpose and assurance.

1. Notice feelings of burden, crisis, nervousness and wanting to avoid an illness situation. Stop. Be in this moment with only what is happening now.

2. Stay aware of self-talk, excuses and reasons to avoid the situation. Let go of future thinking and reliance on past experiences. Talk with others about how you feel.

3. Remember the self-fulfilling prophecy and Nocebo implications of getting life expectancy or prognosis statistics, and strongly consider avoiding them.

4. Learn about this sick person as an individual. Find a "calling" and what feels good in helping long-term. Have faith in your ability to manage your involvement.

5. Don't push too hard. Tend the garden of sickness and healing rather than driving the race car.

6. Offer unsolicited help; get past polite refusals. Start now and small. Help the helpers. Expect to feel impatient or irritated at times when helping.

7. Envision and talk about a healing and peaceful journey to wellness with the sick one. Help reduce their sick prejudices. Praise all the big and little accomplishments.

8. Notice and appreciate the enrichment, wisdom and self-satisfaction gained from helping.

Joseph H. McNolty

CHAPTER V. HELPING

The good that comes from helping a sick person is not just the comple-
tion of tasks, but the more valuable display of caring. Caring isn't just a
fuzzy, soft emotion that doesn't really matter. In fact, the friendship
and affection that comes with caring can mean the difference between
life and death, as seen in "Social Relationships and Mortality Risk:
A Meta-analytic Review."[41] (It also nourishes us in unexpected
ways, as we'll see in the What We Gain section.) For me, it meant
that I wasn't forgotten and there was some understanding of what
I was going through. Even token gestures were deeply meaningful because I knew some of the people didn't have first-hand
experience with a serious illness and for them to be doing something was a warm leap of faith on their part.

PART A. FINDING OUR "CALLING" AS HELPERS

HELPING in ways we feel good about is good "medicine" for them
and us. Just the opposite is true when we feel forced to help for a
long time in ways we don't like. It can create thoughts of sacrifice
in us and feelings of guilt in our sick friend, resulting in an
undertone of resentment in the climate. Helpers should choose
ways to support the sick one that they feel good about. Of course,
at times it's the laundry and dishes that need to be done and
we're the only ones around. Long-term, though, we must make it
more what we want it to be.

An easy way to decide how to help is by clearing the mind
and sitting quietly for at least fifteen minutes. We've already
talked to our sick loved one and understand the questions and
feelings they may have. Remember to consider what may help
the helpers as reasonable ways to contribute. Write down all the
things that can be done for the sick person in the next two weeks
(ten to twenty ideas). Pick those few that give you the best feeling

when you think of doing them. Once you start, they will evolve
and change from month to month, anyway, as you try things. Just
jump in and get something going. Below are some ideas to start
thinking about:

- Taking them to doctor appointments
- Helping with decisions
- Doing laundry
- Getting food for them, organizing meals, or delivering
  dinner once a week
- Taking a child to school
- Walking the dog
- Doing yardwork monthly
- Staying with the sick one and giving a break to the
  main caregiver
- Doing housework (scheduling or paying for a
  housekeeper)
- Assisting with auto maintenance
- Shopping
- Going out to lunch with them regularly
- Paying off some bills
- Coordinating calendars among helpers
- Helping the helpers with their needs

We can bring some settling normalcy into their lives by taking
them to church, out to eat, to play cards with friends, to the
bowling alley, to an AA meeting, or to wherever they are used to
going. Just being there, reading or watching a ballgame together,
can be wonderful support to someone who is sick. It perks up the
atmosphere.

Leaving something on the doorstep is a great thing to do for
both us and the sick one. Often, the sick person doesn't want to
muster the energy to see someone, make themselves look
presentable, and thank them. It's quick for us, too. It can be

arranged with them beforehand or coordinated with other friends who deliver or pick up on other days. A pot of soup is almost always appreciated, as is baked bread. Whatever you're having for dinner can be left for them. If there are dietary restrictions, leave flowers, a book, or a card. Picking up laundry and dropping it off a few days later would be wonderful assistance.

All we need to deal with is what's right in front of us. We don't have to feel like we need to solve all the problems. We're just taking care of a few things this week, enabling the household to keep running, and showing some kindness. If substantial support is needed, contact other friends and family and look into one of the online applications that organize calendars for sick folks and their support people. † These programs are an excellent way to organize and spread tasks out over numerous people.

PART B. OFFERING UNSOLICITED HELP

Our job as helpers is to provide support when it's needed. Some-times our sick friend or loved one can themselves be an obstacle. Customs, reservations, and pride might be getting in the way of their asking for help. We need to *get past their obligatory rejections: "Oh, that's okay," "We'll be fine," "I don't want you to go to any trouble."*

To start, we tell them what we'd like to do, or at least ask about doing the specific ideas we thought about. If they resist, tell them you need to feel like you're doing something to help. Frame the assistance in any way that makes the sick person feel accepted and good about it. Let them know you are there to help. The goal is to just break the ice and get in there to do some things, so that everyone can see how it can work.

Our challenge as helpers is to remain calm and peaceful when we feel those "fight or flight," morose, troubling emotions come on. It takes practice and experience. Seemingly daunting experiences like someone in pain, struggling, or needing to go to the hospital trigger panicky feelings the first few times. I eventu-ally became relatively calm on trips to the emergency room, and would often find time for a nice coffee or meal out when things settled down there. Each time, it would take more to press my "panic button" until I mostly had an inner feeling of quiet. Acceptance and feeling peaceful are obviously good for us, but also reassuring and calming for the sick one when they see us unruffled and smiling. Our relaxed attitude is very good for doctors and nurses to feel settled and keep the mood light for better healing.

From the many, many visits I've made visiting loved ones in hospitals and care facilities, I've found a number of very important ways the patient benefits. First, it's comforting having someone there on many levels for the patient. Second, they can get better care when we ask things of the hospital staff that they may not be able or assertive enough to request. Our presence sends a signal to hospital staff that someone cares about the sick one. This can be like an unwritten currency for more attention. Additionally, an observer there can make for more thorough care as well. It's nice for the hospital staff to get to know family and friends, most of the time.

PART C. DEALING WITH SICK FOLKS WHO ADAMANTLY REFUSE HELP

In tougher cases, the sick person and their family might insist they don't want help. In fact, they may not need any support. That's fine; we can just back off and keep in touch. In other cases, it will be clear they are suffering and are stubborn about receiving help. These folks may act like nothing is wrong. We need to change our approach or back off entirely for a couple of months. In these cases, remain patient and know that this may come from a place of pride, their own assumptions about illness, and not wanting to be a burden.

We can also attempt to couch help in ways that seem like we're doing something already or we enjoy doing it. For example, "The food is left over from dinner and will just go to waste," "I'm going to the store already," or "How about we take the kids for the day? We enjoy them so much." They may just be private and not be feeling presentable, in which case leaving things at the door may work. We can stay alerted to any softening in their position over the weeks and months to come.

PART D. DON'T PUSH TOO HARD

Our fears can cause us to feel desperate to quickly "fix" the sick one. This is especially true in very close relationships. For me, my wife's illness was the most important project there could be. I wasn't going to let anything slip through the cracks or leave any stone unturned in getting her better. I would get into a rigid, task-oriented mode, seamlessly slipping into the fast-paced corporate director I was in my career. I would come up with a blizzard of ideas of what my wife could do next: get even more opinions on a diagnosis, fly to different clinics, make dietary changes, try new medicines, etc. It could wear her out just thinking about it, and me too. Our sick prejudice can lead us to approach the situation with a grim determination that circumvents the good we're trying to achieve.

Our ideas can all be good ones, but there is a pace to things. What is best for the sick one's morale and long-term energy must be balanced with getting results. Pushing hard and bringing feelings of desperation into the situation can obviously be stressful for our loved one, but it can also burn us out in the long run.

As hard as it may be to box the illness in, it needs to be a project and not a life. Our best approach is to keep the pace leisurely, continue to have fun however possible, and let the doctors do their job. Even if the illness is progressing quickly, it's important to pace ourselves. The illness process is more like planting a garden. We give the medicines, treatments, and surgeries time to work at their own pace. Like writing a book or restoring a car, we do a little each day, and the rest is life as usual. Even in cases where the illness is truly chronic and may never get better, the balance needs to be there. My wife's condition the last five years included severe, twenty-four-hour pain that we never found a cure for. We kept checking around, though, trying different things and controlling as much as we could. She was always good about living life as usual and not allowing the illness to stop things she enjoyed and could reasonably do.

CHAPTER VI. MOVING PAST OUR SICK PREJUDICE

As we've seen, our attitudes are based on a mishmash of primordial emotions, sickness stereotypes, TV, sick people in our past, and future thinking, and very little on just this person today. That is a form of bias and prejudiced thinking. When we move past it, we free our sick loved one from the burden of a history that isn't theirs and give them an open future. In the process, we give ourselves wonderful gifts, too.

PART A. WHAT WE GAIN

We realize many short and long-term benefits as we get through our sick prejudice mode. There is great personal growth and wisdom that can come from hardships like illness—which can be attained by helping and not by having to get sick! On the surface, it may appear that we're doing more chores, housework, and errands. There is, however, pure self-satisfaction of assisting an ill person that is valuable in many aspects of our life.

In many ways, an illness can provide a needed turning point in our lives. Stephen Richards said, "When you reach out to those in need, do not be surprised if the essential meaning of something occurs."[42] Illness is a wake-up call to enjoy each moment and resolutely follow our dreams while we can. We don't want to sleep through it. My wife's sickness and my own were certainly wake-up calls for me. *I made changes I had needed for many years but thought they were impossible to make before I was sick: a career change, learning a musical instrument, becoming more spiritual, and having "permission" to do what I enjoyed.*

Right off the bat, when my wife was first getting diagnosed, it was the most stressful, catastrophic period of my life. So many things appeared to be collapsing. In the midst of it, I distinctly remember feeling an overwhelming sense of gratefulness for all that we did have and all that was going well. I believe I had a greater feeling of thankfulness than many other people. *They didn't have the opportunity of having their world shaken to the core to see all that still clung tight.* Nor did they stand to lose so much to be able to see the true value of what they had. Of course, things worked out well in the end and all my turmoil was unneeded. As John Lennon and others said: "Everything will be okay in the end. If it's not okay, it's not the end."

We learn we're much stronger than we thought. It releases the strength of our spirit and brings clarity of purpose. Being around and supporting ill people can be a true fear of ours. It always feels tremendous to conquer a fear. Even more, the greatest stories, dreams, victories, battles, and evidence of human character can be found in times of sickness. If we avoid sickness, we miss that side of our life experience and the satisfaction from providing assistance.

We have an inbred, natural desire to help and care for someone sick that has evolved over millions of years.[43] Because of that, it can give us a unique kind of satisfaction that we would miss in our lives otherwise. It's similar to the good feelings we get from doing a job well or cuddling a baby. It's fulfilling to see the results from helping someone and their family when they're stretched thin.

On the family level and in the small community groups we lived in for most of our evolution, the sick and dying would be near and a part of our daily lives. This makes sickness an integral part of life, not one to be avoided. It shouldn't be considered "sappy," then, to say it is something to be appreciated for the meaning and balance it gives to the rest of our lives. The problem is, then, that we miss out as potential helpers because illness can be hidden and "swept under the rug" in more sickness-averse, aesthetically focused cultures. We as potential helpers then miss out on valuable experiences.

We continually redefine what is actually difficult, bad, urgent, or painful when we spend some time in a sickness situation. For me, the perspective of seeing what is really the "big stuff" and "little stuff" in my life is invaluable. Illness cuts through daily routine and petty irritations, putting into perspective all that we have and hope for. Things we used to think would be dire situations can become part of the "job" as we loosen our expectations. It's settling to be able to remain calm in situations others often find stressful.

PART B. WHAT'S LEFT AFTER A SICK PREJUDICE IS GONE

When a sick prejudice and all its drama is stripped away, there isn't much left. It can seem like something's missing after being hyped-up on primitive emotions. What's happening at any given time with this sick one is probably very little. What we're getting "involved" in is usually very basic. Getting involved a couple of times a week turns out not to be the big deal we envisioned. We start noticing that helping with an illness mostly boils down to some chores, errands, watching TV, and sitting around talking. That, in most cases, helping with a chronic illness is easier than helping someone with the flu.

What we narrowly thought of as lost time from helping, we gained in so many other ways. What we were fighting to save time for in our lives turns out not to be as important as helping, and we enjoy them more after doing meaningful work for someone.

We feel better when we stop dragging around all the negative sick prejudice baggage. We're aware of how quickly our emotions can pull us into the ancient past, and how easily our minds can push us into the distant future. We stay centered and in the moment with our sick friend or family member, where we find it calm and meaningful.

We can be open to all the good that can occur rather than expecting the worst. The cloudy generalizations all clear, and everyone feels brighter. As we let go of our sick prejudices, we can see light in situations that we thought were dark and foreboding. We realize illness is just another side of life to experience, and that it comes and goes. We know we can create ways of helping that work for us.

We don't fear getting stuck in a situation. We know our limits in helping and what to do when we reach them. This, in turn, can enable us to be more giving and sympathetic to others and deactivates our self-centered survival triggers. We're now calmly doing what we can to activate good healing outcomes through the positive environment we create. We're making our experience feel better for us in the process. Finally, we can be fully present as helpers now, and one day as patients ourselves.

RESOURCES

*For more on the emotional stages that people go through during a serious illness, please see following sources.

JoAnn LeMaistre, "Coping With Chronic Illness," adapted from *After The Diagnosis* (Berkeley: Ulysses, 1995), assessed March 24, 2017 http://www.alpineguild.com/COP-ING%20WITH%20CHRONIC%20ILLNESS.html.

Jennifer Martin, "The 7 Psychological Stages of Chronic Pain," The Pain News Network, September 14, 2015, https://www.painnewsnetwork.org/stories/2015/9/13/the-7-psychological-stages-of-chronic-pain-illness

National Cancer Institute, "Feelings & Cancer," December 2, 2014
http://www.cancer.gov/about-cancer/coping/feelings

†Online programs, descriptions and reviews for coordinating
family and friends to help sick people with meals, chores and
appointments.

Jeff Anderson, "Best (and Worst) Apps for Caregivers," *A Place for
Mom,* April 24, 2015, http://www.aplaceformom.com/blog/best-
and-worst-apps-for-caregivers-07-03-2013/

CareCalendar, https://www.carecalendar.org/

END NOTES

1. Brian W. Ward, Jeannine S. Schiller, Richard A. Goodman, "Multiple Chronic Conditions Among US Adults: A 2012 Update," abstract, *Preventing Chronic Disease* 11 (2014), doi: http://dx.doi.org/10.5888/pcd11.130389.

2. National Alliance for Caregiving in collaboration with AARP, "Caregiving in the U.S. 2009" (NAC and AARP, 2009), http://www.caregiving.org/data/Caregiving_in_the_US_2009_full_report.pdf.

3. "Family and Social Support," Baltimore: Johns Hopkins Center to Eliminate Cardiovascular Health Disparities, accessed April 10, 2017, http://www.jhsph.edu/research /centers-and-institutes/johns-hopkins-center-to-eliminate-cardiovascular-health-disparities/about/influencesonhealth/family_social_support.html.

4. Epictetus, ed. Carol Vivyan, "Quotes for Therapy: Epictetus 55–135 AD," GetSelfHelp.co.uk, 2015, https://www.getselfhelp.co.uk/epictetus.htm.

5. Horacio Fábrega, Jr., *Evolution of Sickness and Healing* (Berkley: University of California Press, 1997).

6. Horacio Fábrega, Jr., in conversation with the author, October 2016.

7. K.M. Cohen, S.C. Finney, P.L. Gibbard, and J.X. Fan, "The ICS International Chronostratigraphic Chart," last updated 2013, http://www.stratigraphy.org/ICSchart/ChronostratChart2015-01.pdf.

8. Ellen Castelow, "Disease in Medieval England," *History Magazine,* accessed April 10, 2017, http://www.historic-uk.com/HistoryUK/HistoryofEngland/Disease-in-Medieval-England/.

9. Arizona State University, "Prejudice Is Hard-wired Into The Human Brain, Says ASU Study," abstract, ScienceDaily, May 25, 2005, https://www.sciencedaily.com/releases/2005/05

10. Pamela M. Casey, Roger K. Warren, Fred L. Cheesman II,

and Jennifer K. Elek, "Implicit Bias Frequently Asked Questions," in *Helping Courts Address Implicit Bias: Resources for Education* (National Center for State Courts, 2012), http://www.ncsc.org/~/media/Files/PDF/Topics/Gender%20and%20Racial%20Fairness/IB_report_033012.ashx.

11. Ibid.

12. Horacio Fábrega, Jr., *Evolution of Sickness and Healing* (Berkley: University of California Press, 1997), 216.

13. Ibid., 30.

14. Horacio Fábrega, Jr., *Evolution of Sickness and Healing* (Berkley: University of California Press, 1997) 51; Laurie A. Rudman, "Social Justice in Our Minds, Homes, and Society: The Nature, Causes, and Consequences of Implicit Bias," *Social Justice Research* 17, no. 2 (2004): 129–142, http://rutgerssocialcognitionlab.weebly.com/uploads/1/3/9/7/13979590/rudman2004sjr_1.pdf.

15. "Søren Kierkengaard Quotes," GoodReads Quotable Quote, accessed March 24, 2017, http://www.goodreads.com/quotes/152450-the-most-painful-state-of-being-is-remembering-the-future.

16. U.S. Census Bureau, "U.S. Household Incomes: A Snapshot," Federal Reserve Bank of San Francisco Economic Education & Outreach, last modified October 5, 2015, http://www.census.gov/hhes/www/cpstables/032015/hhinc/hinc01_000.htm.

17. "Multiple Myeloma: Risk Factors," Cancer.Net, last modified October 2016, http://www.cancer.net/cancer-types/multiple-myeloma/risk-factors.

18. H. Ludwig et al, "Myeloma in patients younger than age 50 years presents with more favorable features and shows better survival: an analysis of 10,549 patients from the International Myeloma Working Group," abstract, *Blood* 111, no. 8 (2008), doi 10.1182/blood-2007-03-081018.

19. Katherine S. Tippett and Yasmin S. Cypel, ed. *Design and Operation: The Continuing Survey of Food Intakes by Individuals and*

the Diet and Health Knowledge Survey, 1994–96 (United States Department of Agriculture, 1997).

20. Julianne Holt-Lunstad, Timothy B. Smith, and J. Bradley Layton, "Social Relationships and Mortality Risk: A Meta-analytic Review," PLoS Med 7, no. 7 (2010). doi: 10.1371/journal.pmed.1000316.

21. Ibid.

22. "Medical Definition of Placebo Effect," MedicineNet.com, May 13, 2016, http://www.medicinenet.com/script/main/art.asp?articlekey=31481.

23. Cara Feinberg, "The Placebo Phenomenon: An ingenious researcher finds the real ingredients of 'fake' medicine," Harvard Magazine (January–February 2013), http://harvardmagazine.com/2013/01/the-placebo-phenomenon.

24. WebMD, "What Is the Placebo Effect?" February 23, 2016, http://www.webmd.com/pain-management/what-is-the-placebo-effect#1.

25. Ted J. Kaptchuk and Franklin G Miller, Ph.D., "Placebo Effects in Medicine," *The New England Journal of Medicine* 373 (2015): 8–9, doi: 10.1056/NEJMp1504023.

26. Cara Feinberg, "The Placebo Phenomenon: An ingenious researcher finds the real ingredients of 'fake' medicine," *Harvard Magazine* (January–February 2013), http://harvardmagazine.com/2013/01/the-placebo-phenomenon.

27. Lissa Rankin, "The Nocebo Effect: Negative Thoughts Can Harm Your Health," *Psychology Today,* August 6, 2013, https://www.psychologytoday.com/blog/owning-pink/201308/the-nocebo-effect-negative-thoughts-can-harm-your-health.

28. Kaada B., "Tidsskr Nor Laegeforen" [Nocebo—the opposite of placebo], PMC 109, no. 7-8 (1989): 814–821, http://www.ncbi.nlm.nih.gov/pubmed/2650014.

29. Cara Feinberg, "The Placebo Phenomenon: An ingenious researcher finds the real ingredients of 'fake' medicine," *Harvard*

Magazine (January–February 2013), http://harvardmagazine.-com/2013/01/the-placebo-phenomenon.

30. Massachusetts General Hospital, "Study confirms impact of clinician-patient relationship on health outcomes," Mass General News, news release, April 9, 2014, http://www.massgeneral.org/about/pressrelease.aspx?id=1691.

31. Mary Morrisey, "Week 2, Making Money Welcome," *Prosperity Plus II: Harnessing Your Invisible Power* (Simi Valley, CA: LifeSOULutions That Work, LLC, 2013–2016), DVD.

32. Ibid.

33. Cara Feinberg, "The Placebo Phenomenon: An ingenious researcher finds the real ingredients of 'fake' medicine," *Harvard Magazine* (January–February 2013), http://harvardmagazine.-com/2013/01/the-placebo-phenomenon.

34. Keith J. Petrie and John Weinman, *Perceptions of Health and Illness: Current Research and Applications* (Milton, UK: Taylor & Francis, 1997).

35. Horacio Fábrega, Jr., *Evolution of Sickness and Healing* (Berkley: University of California Press, 1997).

36. Ibid., 34.

37. Gordon B. Hinckley, *Standing for Something: 10 Neglected Virtues That Will Heal Our Hearts and Homes* (New York: Harmony, 2001), 86.

38. Eckhart Tolle, *The Power of Now* (Vancouver, BC: Namaste Publishing, 2004), 43.

39. Horacio Fábrega, Jr., *Evolution of Sickness and Healing* (Berkley: University of California Press, 1997), 92.

40. Shannon L. Alder, GoodReads Quotable Quote, accessed May 3, 2017, https://www.goodreads.com/quotes/7365095-one-of-the-most-important-things-you-can-do-on

41. Julianne Holt-Lunstad, Timothy B. Smith, and J. Bradley Layton, "Social Relationships and Mortality Risk: A Meta-analytic Review," PLoS Med 7, no. 7 (2010). doi: 10.1371/journal.pmed.1000316.

42. Stephen Richards, GoodReads Quotable Quote, accessed May 3, 2017, https://www.goodreads.com/quotes/540266-when-you-reach-out-to-those-in-need-do-not

43. Horacio Fábrega, Jr., *Evolution of Sickness and Healing* (Berkley: University of California Press, 1997), 29–34.